The 15-D Detox Plan: Lose Weight, Boost Energy & Rejuvenate Your Skin Naturally

A Full-Body Reset for Fast Fat Loss, Glowing Skin & Anti-Aging – Easy Recipes & Supplements to Transform Your Health

◆ ◆ ◆

Gregory Long

Copyright © 2025 by Gregory Long

ISBN 979-8-3090998-9-4

First printing 2025
Printed and bound in the United States of America.

All rights reserved.

No part of this publication may be reproduced, stored in a retrieval system, or transmitted in any form or by any means, electronic, mechanical, photocopying, recording or otherwise, without written permission of the Publisher. For information from the Publisher about permissions, excerpts, options and other permission(s), submit written requests to: StartYourDetox@gmail.com

Disclaimer

The author of this book does not dispense medical advice or prescribe the use of any technique as a form of treatment for physical, emotional, or medical problems without the advice of a physician, either directly or indirectly. The intent of the author is to only offer information of a general nature to help you in your quest for emotional, physical, and spiritual well-being. In the event you use any of the information in this book for yourself, the author and the publisher assume no responsibility for your actions.

Table Of Contents

Introduction: Welcome To Your Full Body Reset 5

Chapter 1: The Fab 5 – Your Powerhouse Supplements 8

Chapter 2: Wellness Upgrades 16

Chapter 3: Grocery List & Kitchen Essentials 23

Chapter 4: Daily Schedule – Reset and Refresh 27

Chapter 5: 15-Day Meal Plan & Recipes 35

Chapter 6: Post-Detox Maintenance & Lifestyle Plan 70

Chapter 7: Healing Recipes for Vitamin & Mineral Deficiencies
& Common Health Concerns 76

Chapter 8: Closing Remarks & Gratitude 83

بسم الله الرحمن الرحيم

INTRODUCTION

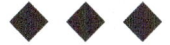

Welcome To Your Full Body Reset

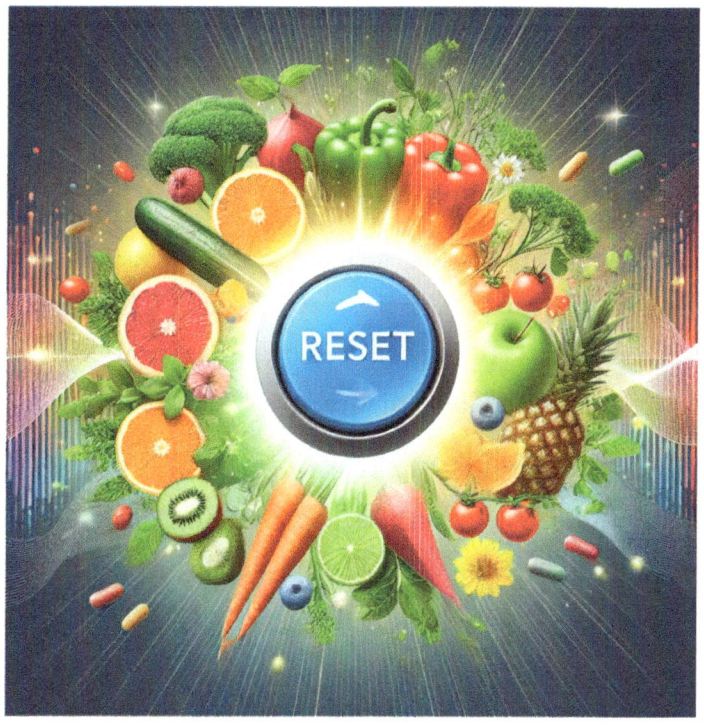

Are you tired of feeling sluggish, weighed down, and disconnected from the vibrant, energetic version of yourself? Have you tried diet after diet, only to see the weight creep back while your cravings, fatigue, and bloating refuse to disappear?

If you're reading this, you're ready for real change. Not a quick fix. Not another fad. But a true reset—a transformation that works from the inside out, helping you shed excess weight, increase your energy, clear your skin, and feel ageless in just 15 days.

This program is designed to do what no other detox can—help you unlock your body's natural ability to burn fat, repair itself, and thrive. No starvation. No extreme restrictions. Just powerful, nutrient-dense foods and supplements that work with your body to eliminate what's been holding you back.

Why This Works When Nothing Else Has

Traditional diets fail because they focus on restriction instead of restoration. Your body isn't designed to be at war with itself. When given the right tools—the right foods, the right supplements, and the right timing—it naturally burns fat, balances hormones, clears inflammation, and restores your youthful energy.

This Full Body Reset is based on a strategic combination of five powerhouse supplements (The Fab 5), nourishing whole foods, and a daily rhythm that syncs with your body's natural detoxification cycles.

Most people lose 8-12 pounds in 15 days while experiencing:

- Effortless fat loss without extreme workouts or calorie counting
- Glowing, even-toned skin as your body clears inflammation from within

- Unstoppable energy from morning to night
- Balanced digestion—say goodbye to bloating, constipation, and sluggish metabolism
- Sharper focus and a clear mind as brain fog disappears

What To Expect In The Next 15 Days

For the next two weeks, your body will go through an incredible transformation. You'll experience a rapid shift as toxins, excess fat, and built-up waste are eliminated, leaving you lighter, clearer, and more vibrant than ever.

This book will guide you through:

- The Fab 5 Supplements—a game-changer in fat loss, energy, and skin renewal
- A simple daily routine designed for maximum results
- Delicious, satisfying meals that heal your body while keeping you full
- The ultimate maintenance plan so your results last a lifetime

By the end of these 15 days, you'll feel completely different—inside and out. This is the beginning of a new era of health, confidence, and vitality.

Are you ready to reset your body, reclaim your energy, and step into the best version of yourself?

Let's get started!

CHAPTER 1

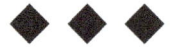

The Fab 5 – Your Powerhouse Supplements

The Secret to Effortless Weight Loss, Glowing Skin, and Endless Energy

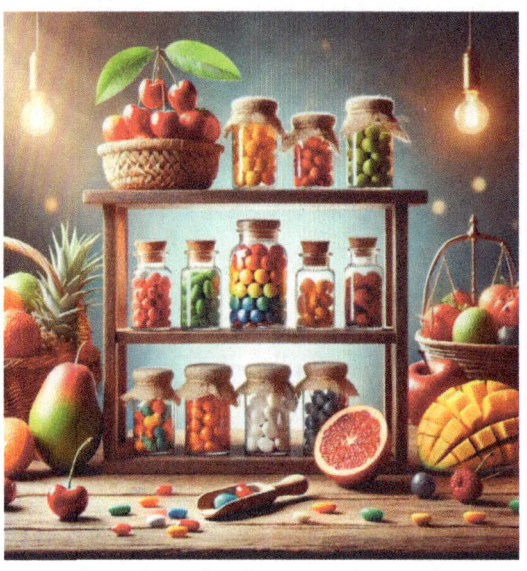

Most detox programs fail because they focus only on elimination—cutting out foods, counting calories, or drinking bland green juices. But true transformation isn't just about what you take out—it's about what you put in. Your body is designed to heal, burn fat, and thrive, but it needs the right fuel to do so.

That's where The Fab 5 comes in.

These five powerhouse supplements are the key to unlocking your body's full potential—helping you burn stubborn fat, eliminate toxins, and restore balance at a cellular level. They work synergistically to supercharge your metabolism, increase energy, clear inflammation, and even improve brain function—all while making weight loss feel effortless.

The results? Life-changing. Jaw-dropping. Absolutely undeniable.

Thousands of people have already transformed their bodies and lives using The Fab 5, and the reviews speak for themselves.

"I lost 10 pounds in the first week, and I wasn't even hungry. My cravings disappeared so fast!"

"I used to wake up exhausted every day. Now, I have energy from morning to night without even needing coffee!"

"My skin has NEVER looked this good. People keep asking what I'm doing!"

You can get all five supplements exclusively at www.heycoachgreg.com.

Now, let's break down each one:

1. High School Skinny – The Fat Burner Craving Crusher

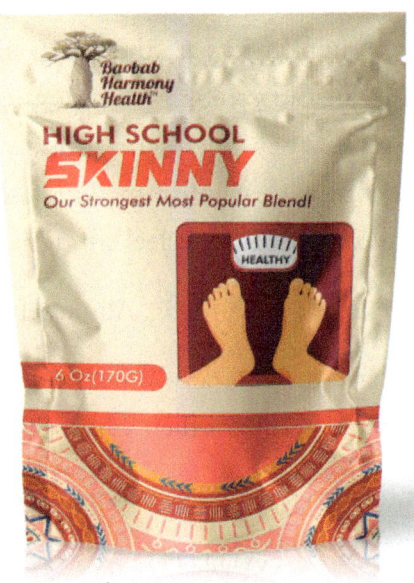

This is the game-changer for people who have struggled with belly fat, emotional eating, and sugar cravings. High School Skinny naturally reprograms your metabolism, melting stubborn fat while eliminating those relentless cravings for junk food.

- Jaw-Dropping Reviews: www.heycoachgreg.com

"This is the only thing that ever stopped my sugar cravings. I don't even want junk food anymore!"

"I lost inches off my waist without even trying. My stomach is the flattest it's ever been!"

"I feel like I rewound time. I have the same energy and body I had in high school!"

2. Blue Shield – The Inflammation Fighter & Circulation Booster

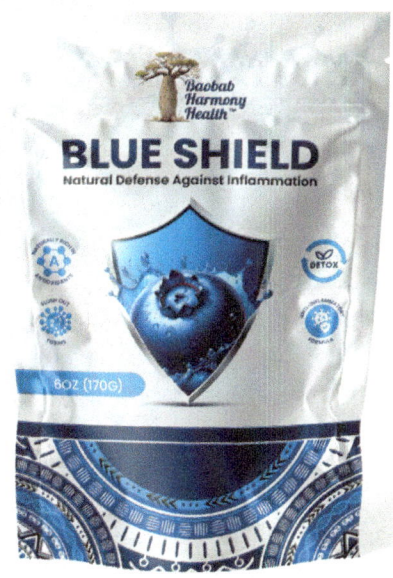

If you have joint pain, sluggish circulation, or feel like your body is constantly inflamed, Blue Shield is your answer. It flushes inflammation from the body, strengthens joints, and restores blood flow, so you feel lighter, more mobile, and pain-free.

- Jaw-Dropping Reviews: www.heycoachgreg.com

"I used to have freezing hands and feet all the time. Now, they're warm again—my circulation is back!"

"My joints don't ache anymore. I can move like I did in my 20s!"

"I had constant mucus and sinus congestion for years. Blue Shield cleared it up in DAYS!"

3. Full Battery – The Energy Restorer & Metabolism Enhancer

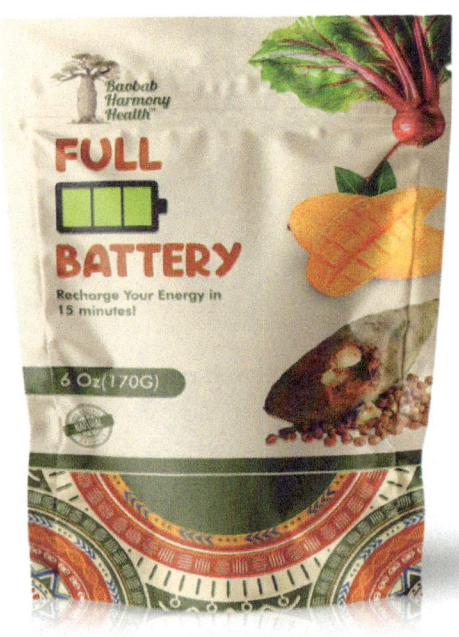

Feeling exhausted every day? Full Battery recharges your body at a cellular level, giving you sustained, all-day energy without caffeine crashes. Wake up refreshed, stay focused, and power through your day effortlessly.

- Jaw-Dropping Reviews: www.heycoachgreg.com

"I was addicted to coffee—until Full Battery. Now I wake up refreshed and energized naturally!"

"No more 3 PM crashes. My energy is stable from morning to night!"

"My workouts are stronger, I feel more motivated, and I'm actually getting things DONE!"

4. Stress Free Genius – The Brain & Nervous System Reset

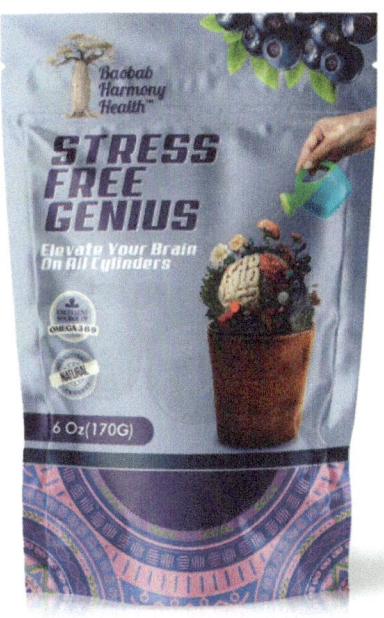

Stress wreaks havoc on the body, causing weight gain, brain fog, and poor sleep. Stress Free Genius is a total reset for your nervous system, calming the mind while enhancing focus, memory, and deep sleep.

- Jaw-Dropping Reviews: www.heycoachgreg.com

"I finally sleep through the night. My mind is calm, and I wake up feeling amazing!"

"I used to have constant anxiety. Now, I feel clear, focused, and relaxed all day."

"The mental clarity is unreal. I can focus better at work, and my thoughts are finally sharp!"

5. Green Multi - The Nutrient Powerhouse for Whole-Body Support

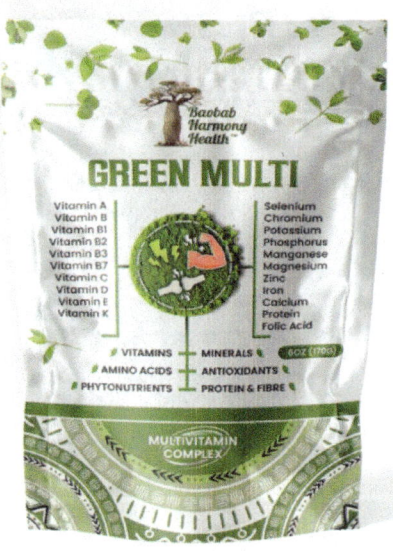

Nutrient deficiencies slow down weight loss, weaken the immune system, and cause muscle and joint pain. Green Multi floods your body with essential vitamins, minerals, and plant-based protein, keeping your body strong, lean, and resilient.

- Jaw-Dropping Reviews: www.heycoachgreg.com

"My joint pain is GONE. I can actually run and exercise without feeling stiff!"

"I didn't realize how nutrient-deficient I was. My skin is clearer, my energy is better, and my digestion has improved!"

"This should be called 'super fuel'—it makes my whole body feel alive!"

Where to Get The Fab 5

These supplements have transformed thousands of lives and they're only available at www.heycoachgreg.com.

If you're ready to experience the same jaw-dropping transformation, order your Fab 5 today and start your 15-Day Reset.

Now that you know the secret weapon behind this program, let's dive into the 15-Day Detox Plan and how to make this transformation effortless!

CHAPTER 2

Wellness Upgrades

Elevate Your Health Beyond The Reset

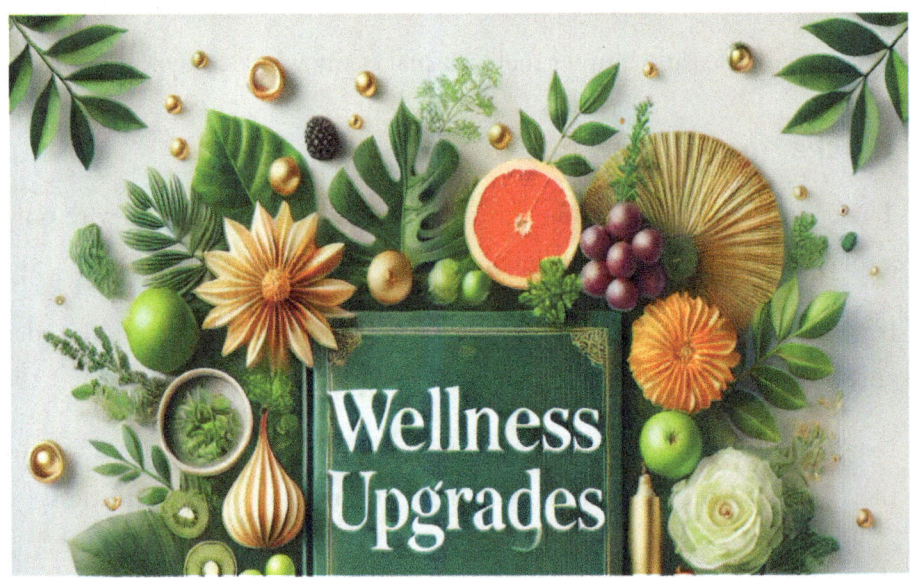

Optimizing Your Health with Targeted Support

While the Full Body Reset lays the foundation for transformation, some individuals may need additional support to address specific health concerns. That's where the Wellness Upgrades come in.

These optional but highly effective supplements help tackle common health issues such as:

- Blood pressure imbalances
- Skin concerns like hyperpigmentation & eczema
- Hair thinning or slow growth
- Muscle fatigue & nutrient deficiencies

By incorporating targeted nutrition & supplementation, you can take your results to the next level and continue improving your health long after the 15 days.

The 4 Wellness Upgrades & Their Benefits

Each of these Wellness Upgrades is designed to work synergistically with the Fab 5 supplements while addressing deeper health concerns.

1. Pressure Balance – Naturally Lower Blood Pressure in 5 Days

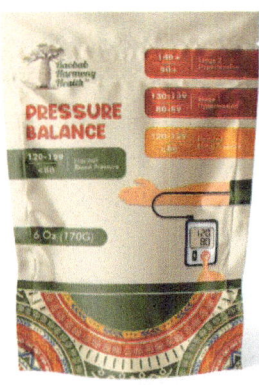

Who It's For: Anyone dealing with high blood pressure or taking medication to regulate it.

Key Benefits:

- Lowers blood pressure naturally without medication.
- Improves circulation & heart function.
- Relieves headaches & stress-related hypertension.
- Supports kidney health & reduces water retention.

How to Use:

Take 1 tablespoon of Pressure Balance with a morning smoothie or juice.

- Best paired with: Full Battery for an energy boost without raising blood pressure.

- Jaw-Dropping Results: Many users report normal blood pressure readings by Day 6 and are able to reduce or eliminate medication within weeks!

2. EvenTone Skin – Achieve Clear, Even-Toned & Glowing Skin

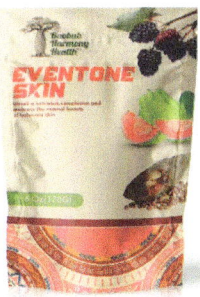

Who It's For: Anyone dealing with dark spots, hyperpigmentation, eczema, psoriasis, or uneven skin tone.

Key Benefits:

- Evens skin tone & fades hyperpigmentation.
- Reduces breakouts, rashes, & skin inflammation.
- Repairs skin from within, leading to a glow by Day 5.
- Regulates body temperature (helps with night sweats & cold hands/feet).

How to Use:

Take 1 tablespoon with High School Skinny or Take 1 tablespoon at 4:30 PM in one of the following ways:

- With a juicer: Mix with apple, grape, cucumber, and mint juice.
- Without a juicer: Mix with pineapple juice (not from concentrate).
- Jaw-Dropping Results: Users consistently see brighter, clearer skin in just 5 days!

3. Hair Food – Strengthen & Accelerate Hair Growth

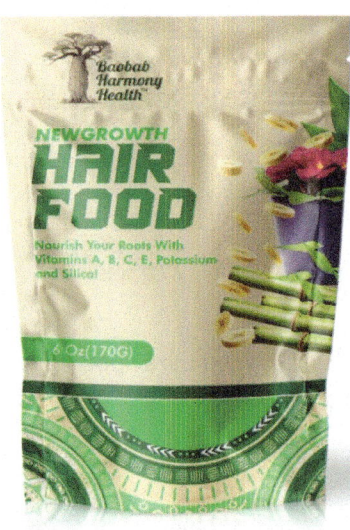

Who It's For: Anyone struggling with thinning hair, slow hair growth, or weak/brittle hair.

Key Benefits:

- Speeds up hair growth & strengthens hair follicles.
- Reduces hair shedding & breakage.
- Increases thickness & volume over time.
- Nourishes the scalp & prevents dandruff.

How to Use:

Take 1 tablespoon daily in a smoothie, juice, or water.

- Best paired with: Green Multi for a complete vitamin boost.
- Jaw-Dropping Results: Users often see baby hairs growing back within 2 weeks and thicker, stronger hair in just 30 days!

4. Milk Silk Cream - Instant Skin Repair & Hydration

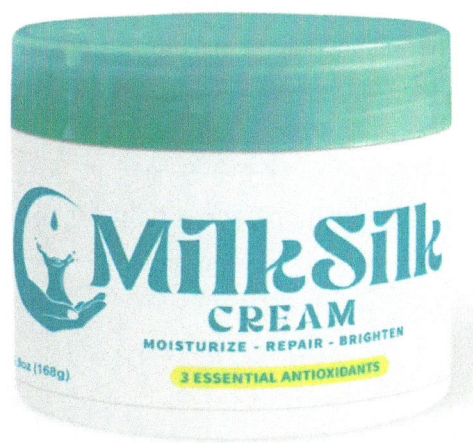

Who It's For: Anyone dealing with dry skin, scars, rashes, burns, or eczema.

Key Benefits:

- Moisturizes & hydrates skin instantly.
- Speeds up wound healing (cuts, burns, scars, and stretch marks).
- Clears rashes, breakouts, & skin irritation overnight.
- Softens rough patches & prevents dryness.

How to Use:

Apply a small amount to any part of the body, including the face.

- Best used: At night before bed for overnight repair.
- Jaw-Dropping Results: Visible improvement overnight and completely healed skin within days!

Final Thoughts: Elevate Your Health

These Wellness Upgrades give you the option to go even further with your transformation. Whether it's balancing blood pressure, achieving glowing skin, strengthening hair, or repairing skin issues, these additions ensure your results last beyond 15 days.

- If you're unsure which upgrade is right for you, reach out to Coach Greg for personalized guidance at startyourdetox@gmail.com

CHAPTER 3

Grocery List & Kitchen Essentials

How to Shop Smart for the Full Body Reset

The Full Body Reset Program is designed to be cost-effective, practical, and easy to follow. This updated grocery list includes ONLY the ingredients used in the 15 meals and adjusts portion sizes to reduce costs while ensuring you have enough for 15 days.

At the end of this chapter, we'll also cover why certain foods like dairy, eggs, and starches are excluded and how they'll be reintroduced during the maintenance phase.

Proteins (Per Person)

- Halal Ground Lamb – 2 pounds (for lamb patties and spiced dishes)
- Halal Chicken Thighs – 8 pieces (skin removed or buy skinless to save time)
- Wild-Caught Salmon – 4 fillets (6 ounces each)
- Wild-Caught Cod – 3 fillets (6 ounces each)
- Wild-Caught Mahi-Mahi – 2 fillets (6 ounces each)

Vegetables (Per Person)

- Green Beans – 2 pounds
- Brussels Sprouts – 1.5 pounds
- Chinese Eggplant – 3 medium-sized
- Romaine Lettuce – 2 heads
- Kale – 2 bunches
- Spinach – 2 bunches
- Red Cabbage – 1 head
- Bell Peppers – 4 (2 red, 2 yellow)
- Zucchini – 3 medium-sized
- Broccoli – 2 heads
- Cauliflower – 1 head
- Cucumbers – 4 large
- Cherry Tomatoes – 2 pints
- Onions (Red, White, or Yellow) – 2 pounds
- Fresh Garlic – 2 bulbs

Fruits (Per Person)

- Fresh Apples (Fuji, Gala, or Pink Lady) – 10 apples
- Frozen Dark Sweet Cherries – 2.5 pounds
- Frozen Pineapples – 2 pounds
- Frozen Mangoes – 2 pounds

Spices & Seasonings

To keep costs low, only the spices used in the recipes are included:

- Himalayan Salt – 1 container (8 ounces)
- Garlic Powder – 1 container
- Onion Powder – 1 container
- Smoked Paprika – 1 container
- Cumin Powder – 1 container
- Turmeric Powder – 1 container
- Black Pepper – 1 container
- Crushed Red Pepper Flakes – 1 container
- Dried Oregano – 1 container
- Ground Coriander – 1 container
- Italian Seasoning – 1 container
- Fresh Dill – 1 bunch
- Curry Powder – 1 container
- Ground Cinnamon – 1 container (for smoothies and dressings)
- Fresh Mint Leaves – 1 bunch

Cooking Oils & Condiments

- Avocado Oil (for Cooking) – 1 bottle (16 ounces)
- Olive Oil (for Dressings & Sauces) – 1 bottle (16 ounces)
- Dijon Mustard – 1 small jar (for dressings and sauces)
- Tahini – 1 small jar (for tahini drizzle in recipes)

Kitchen Tools

- Blender – Essential for smoothies, dressings, and sauces.
- Measuring Spoons – Ensures accurate spice and supplement measurements.

- Cold-Pressed Juicer (Optional) – For fresh, nutrient-rich juices.
- Non-Stick Baking Sheets – For roasting proteins and vegetables.
- Sharp Knives – For prepping vegetables and meats efficiently.

Why No Dairy, Eggs, or Starch Products?

This program is designed to detoxify and reset your body by eliminating foods that may slow or hinder the process.

- Dairy – Often causes inflammation, mucus buildup, and digestive issues.
- Eggs – Removed to reduce cholesterol and avoid common allergens.
- Starch Products (Bread, Pasta, Potatoes, Rice, etc.) – Excluded because they:

    Increase constipation and digestive sluggishness
    Raise blood sugar levels if not consumed in moderation
    Contribute to weight gain and water retention

Budget-Saving Tips for Grocery Shopping

- Buy in bulk – Frozen fruits and proteins often cost less when purchased in bulk.
- Choose seasonal produce – Vegetables in season are cheaper and fresher.
- Use store-brand options – Many store-brand spices, oils, and condiments are just as high-quality but cost less.

CHAPTER 4

Daily Schedule – Reset and Refresh

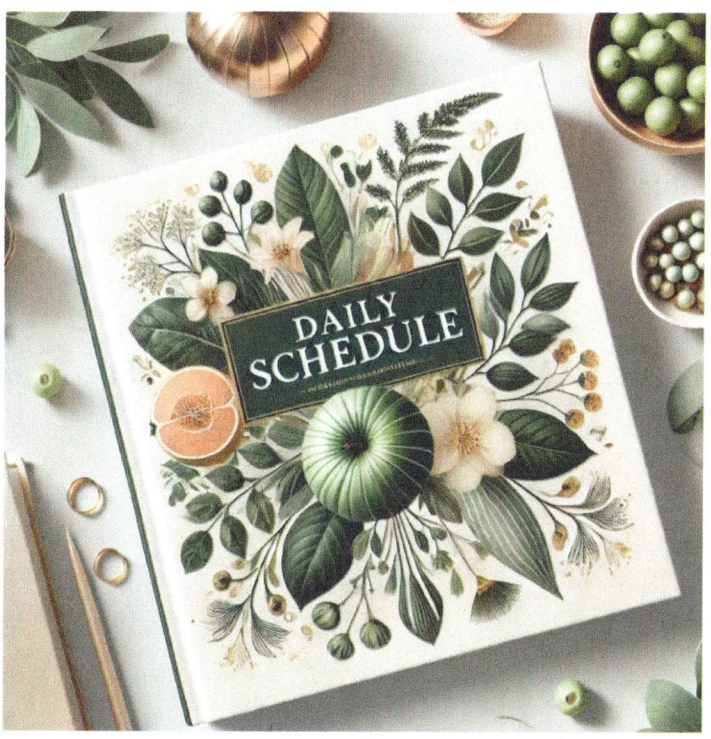

This structured daily plan ensures that your body stays in fat-burning mode, nourished, and energized while detoxing. Each meal, smoothie, and drink has a specific purpose—whether it's to boost metabolism, crush cravings, or enhance digestion and recovery.

However, it's important to listen to your body.

- Meals are optional – If you're not hungry, don't force yourself to eat. The drinks and smoothies provide plenty of nutrients, and forcing extra meals could slow digestion.
- Avoid overeating or overdrinking – This program is about resetting your body, not overwhelming it. If you feel full, you can skip a meal or reduce portion sizes.
- Follow your body's cues – If you miss a scheduled drink or meal, simply pick up where you left off—there's no need to stress or overcompensate.

If you run into scheduling conflicts or need additional support, reach out to Coach Greg at startyourdetox@gmail.com

Morning Smoothie (8:00 AM - 9:00 AM) – Energy & Fat Burning

This smoothie kick starts your metabolism and provides clean, sustained energy to start the day.

Ingredients:

- 2 cups spring water
- 2 cups frozen dark sweet cherries (for antioxidants & digestion support)
- 1 tablespoon Full Battery (for sustained energy & metabolism boost)

Optional Wellness Upgrade: Add 1 tablespoon of Pressure Balance

Directions:

- Add all ingredients to a blender.
- Blend until smooth and creamy.
- our and drink 2 cups.

- ❖ Activates fat-burning mode for the entire day
- ❖ Prevents sugar cravings & hunger crashes
- ❖ Supports brain function & mental clarity

Feeling full from the previous night? If you're not hungry in the morning, you can drink just half the smoothie or skip it entirely.

Brunch Cravings Drink (10:00 AM - 10:30 AM) - Craving Control & Metabolism Support

This drink eliminates sugar cravings and keeps you full until lunch without spiking blood sugar.

Choose ONE of the following options:

Regular Juice Option:

- 1 cup 100% pure apple juice (not from concentrate) OR unfiltered apple juice
- 1 tablespoon High School Skinny (reduces cravings & burns belly fat)

Optional Wellness Upgrade: Add 1 tablespoon of EvenTone Skin

Juicing Options (For Fresh Juice Users)

Apple Cucumber Mint Juice:

- 2 medium apples (Fuji, Gala, or Pink Lady)
- ½ medium cucumber (for hydration & digestion support)
- 6 fresh mint leaves (soothes digestion & refreshes the body)

Apple Pineapple Ginger Juice:

- 1 medium apple
- ½ cup fresh pineapple chunks (for digestion & skin health)
- 1-inch piece fresh ginger (for metabolism & inflammation support)

Directions for Juicing Options:

- Wash and chop all ingredients. Peel the ginger if needed.
- Add ingredients to a juicer and extract juice.
- Measure out 1 cup and drink.

❖ Balances blood sugar & prevents energy crashes
❖ Keeps you full and satisfied
❖ Boosts metabolism & eliminates cravings

Feeling satisfied from your morning smoothie? You can drink half a serving or skip it if not needed.

Lunch (12:00 PM - 1:00 PM) - Nourishment & Fat Loss

Lunch is optional, especially if you're still feeling full from the morning drinks.

- If hungry, have a protein-rich meal with greens to fuel the body.

- If not hungry, skip lunch and go straight to the afternoon drink.

(Lunch Recipes Provided in Chapter 5)

- Supports lean muscle growth & fat burning
- Provides sustained energy & prevents mid-day crashes
- Keeps you full without bloating

Afternoon Immune Drink (2:30 PM - 3:30 PM) - Detox & Inflammation Reduction

This drink helps flush out toxins and reduce inflammation while boosting immunity.

Choose one of the following drinks:

Regular Juice Option:

- 1 cup 100% pure apple juice or 100% pineapple juice (not from concentrate)

Juicing Options (For Fresh Juice Users)

ABC Juice: (Apple, Beet, Carrot)

- 1 medium apple
- 1 small beet (liver detox support & circulation booster)
- 1 medium carrot (rich in vitamins for skin health & digestion)

Seeded Watermelon Juice (Option to Include the Rind):

- 1 cup seeded watermelon chunks (hydration & electrolyte balance)

Apple Pineapple Ginger Juice:

- 1 medium apple
- ½ cup fresh pineapple chunks
- 1-inch piece fresh ginger (gut health & metabolism support)

Directions for Juicing Options:

- Wash and chop all ingredients. Peel the ginger if needed.
- Add ingredients to a juicer and extract juice.
- Measure out 1 cup and drink.

- ❖ Reduces bloating & flushes out toxins
- ❖ Enhances digestion & hydration
- ❖ Boosts skin health & immune system

Supplements: Stir 1 tablespoon of Blue Shield + 1 tablespoon of Green Multi into your chosen juice and drink.

Optional Wellness Upgrade: Add 1 tablespoon of Hair Food

Dinner (5:30 PM - 6:45 PM) - Light, Satisfying, & Restorative

Dinner should be light yet satisfying, providing anti-inflammatory, nutrient-dense foods that aid in overnight detox & repair.

(Dinner Recipes Provided in Chapter 5)

Not very hungry? Reduce your portion size or skip dinner entirely if your body feels satisfied.

- Prepares the body for deep, restorative sleep

- Supports muscle recovery & reduces inflammation
- Prevents late-night cravings & overeating

Night-Time Smoothie (8:00 PM) - Relaxation & Sleep Support

This smoothie calms the nervous system, reduces stress, and promotes deep sleep while continuing the fat-burning process overnight.

Ingredients:

- 1 cup spring water
- 2 cups frozen dark sweet cherries (melatonin-rich for sleep support)
- 1 tablespoon Stress Free Genius (relaxes the brain & nervous system)

Directions:

- Add all ingredients to a blender.
- Blend until smooth.
- Pour and drink 1 cup.

- ❖ Promotes REM sleep for deep recovery
- ❖ Reduces stress & balances cortisol (stress hormone)
- ❖ Continues overnight detox & metabolism support

Not hungry for smoothie? Drink only half or skip it if you don't feel the need for it.

Final Notes: Listen to Your Body

- Don't force meals or drinks—eat only when hungry.

- If your body feels full, skip a meal and continue with the plan as normal.
- If you need additional support or have scheduling conflicts, email Coach Greg at startyourdetox@gmail.com

What's Next?

Now that you have the exact daily schedule, let's move to Chapter 5, where you'll get detailed meal plans & recipes for lunch and dinner to complete the Full Body Reset!

Turn the page to Chapter 5: 15-Day Meal Plan & Recipes!

CHAPTER 5

15-Day Meal Plan & Recipes

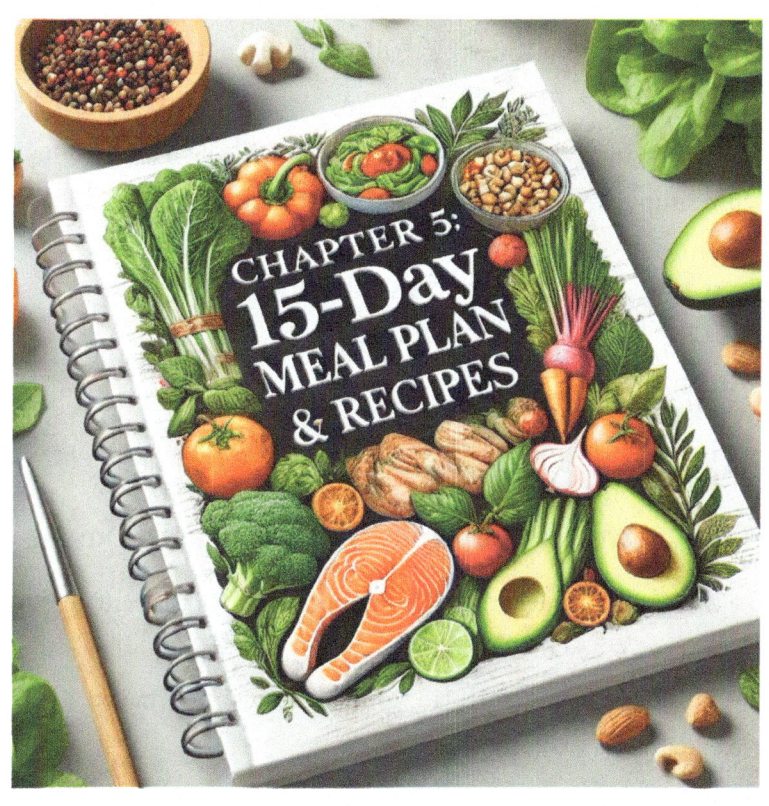

How to Fuel Your Detox for Maximum Results

Now that you have your daily schedule in place, it's time to focus on the solid meals that will nourish your body, keep you satisfied, and maximize fat loss and detoxification.

This meal plan is structured to:

- Keep digestion light while providing essential nutrients.
- Enhance fat-burning by balancing proteins, greens, and anti-inflammatory foods.
- Ensure you feel full and energized without bloating or sluggishness.
- Be simple, budget-friendly, and easy to follow.

Encouragement for Sudden Changes

Flexibility is part of life. Instead of stressing over a missed meal or drink, focus on making the best possible choices with what you have. This program is about building habits that align with your goals. You've got this.

Trust Your Inner Chef (and Forget Cheat Days!)

Let's set the record straight: the dining out tips aren't meant to encourage you to eat out—they're your backup plan, not your go-to option. This program is designed to transform your kitchen into a haven of flavorful, health-packed meals.

Cheat days? Who needs them? With these delicious, saucy, and satisfying recipes, you won't feel deprived. Your taste buds are getting a reset, so junk food won't even tempt you.

The nutrient-packed meals and drinks in this program will leave you so satisfied that even the idea of cheating will feel unnecessary.

By the end of this program, you might just discover a hidden talent for cooking. You'll be blending, sautéing, and seasoning like a pro.

Embrace your inner chef—it's about to shine!

How to Properly Clean Your Meat & Vegetables

Before cooking, it's essential to properly clean your meats and vegetables to remove impurities, bacteria, and residue.

Cleaning Meat with Apple Cider Vinegar or Lemon Juice

- Removes bacteria & excess blood – Natural disinfectants help keep your protein clean.
- Eliminates strong odors – Helps remove the "gamey" smell from poultry, lamb, and seafood.
- Tenderizes the meat – The acidity softens protein fibers, making meat juicier.

Steps to Clean Meat:

- Fill a bowl with cool water (enough to fully submerge the meat).
- Add 1 tablespoon of sea salt to the water.
- Squeeze in the juice of 1 fresh lemon (or use 2 tablespoons of apple cider vinegar).
- Soak the meat for 10–15 minutes (especially for chicken, lamb, and seafood).
- Rinse thoroughly with fresh water before seasoning and cooking.

For tougher meats like lamb or beef, soak in vinegar water for 10 minutes, then give it a final rinse with sea salt and lemon juice for extra freshness.

Cleaning Vegetables for Pesticide Removal

- Removes dirt & chemicals – Helps eliminate wax coatings and pesticide residue.
- Kills bacteria – Especially important for leafy greens and raw vegetables.
- Enhances flavor – Fresh, clean vegetables taste better and absorb seasonings well.

Steps to Clean Vegetables:

- Fill a bowl with water and add 1 tablespoon of apple cider vinegar OR lemon juice.
- Submerge vegetables for 5–10 minutes.
- Rinse thoroughly under fresh running water.
- Pat dry with a clean towel before cooking or storing.

Leafy greens (kale, spinach, romaine) should be soaked and then spun dry.

15 Nourishing & Delicious Meal Options

Pick any meal for lunch or dinner each day based on what sounds good to you!

Each meal includes full seasoning instructions, sauce preparation, and cooking techniques for the best flavors!

1. Zesty Herb-Roasted Chicken Thighs with Lemon-Dill Sauce

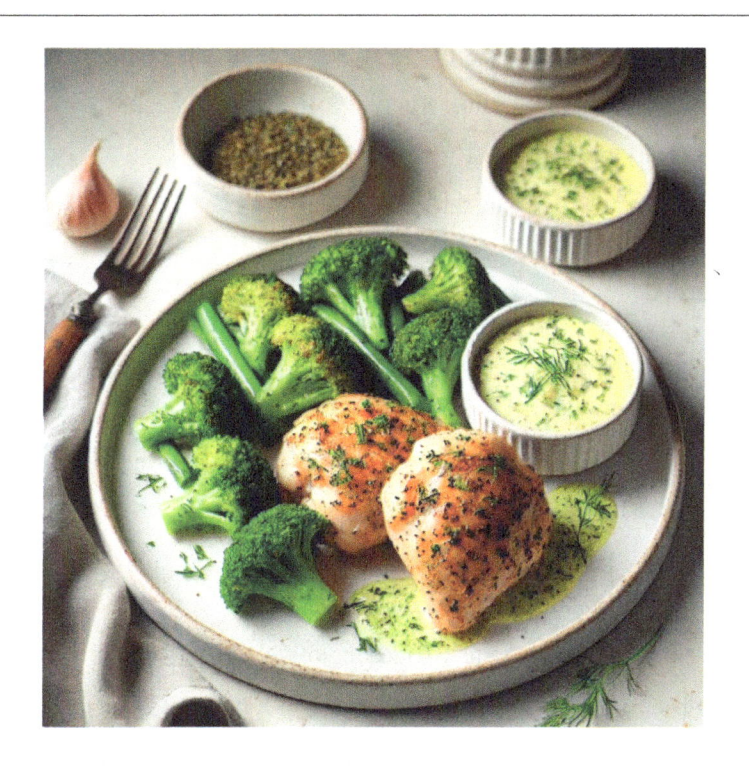

Ingredients:

- 2 chicken thighs (halal optional, skin removed or buy skinless to save time)
- 1 cup steamed broccoli
- 1 tablespoon avocado oil
- ½ teaspoon garlic powder
- ½ teaspoon smoked paprika
- ¼ teaspoon cayenne pepper (optional, for heat)

- ½ teaspoon Himalayan salt

For Lemon-Dill Sauce:

- 1 tablespoon olive oil (not heated, for sauce)
- 1 teaspoon fresh lemon juice
- ½ teaspoon dried dill
- Pinch of Himalayan salt

Directions:

- Preheat the oven to 375°F.
- Pat the chicken dry and rub with garlic powder, smoked paprika, cayenne pepper, and Himalayan salt for a deep, flavorful seasoning.
- Place the chicken thighs on a baking sheet and bake for 25–30 minutes until golden and crispy.
- Steam broccoli for 5 minutes until tender.
- In a small bowl, whisk together olive oil, fresh lemon juice, dried dill, and a pinch of Himalayan salt for the sauce.
- Drizzle the sauce over the roasted chicken before serving.

2. Garlic Lemon Cod with Sautéed Zucchini and Cherry Tomato Medley

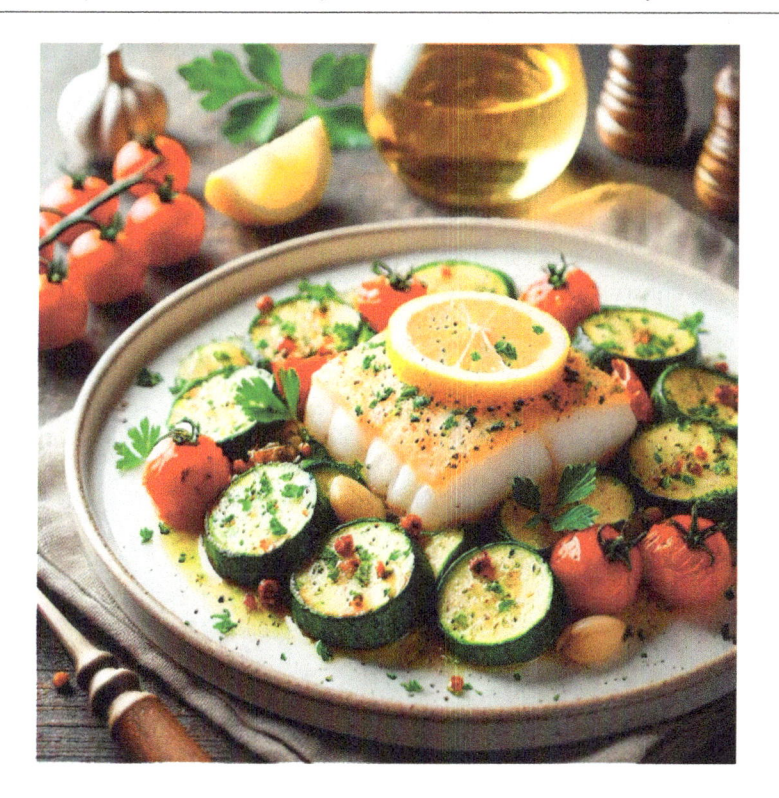

Ingredients:

- 1 wild-caught cod fillet
- 1 cup zucchini slices
- ½ cup cherry tomatoes (halved)
- 1 tablespoon avocado oil
- ½ teaspoon garlic powder
- ½ teaspoon Himalayan salt

- Juice of ½ lemon

Directions:

- Preheat the oven to 375°F.
- Pat the fillet dry and coat with garlic powder and Himalayan salt for a light but flavorful seasoning.
- Place on a baking sheet and bake for 12–15 minutes until flaky.
- Heat avocado oil in a skillet over medium heat. Add zucchini slices and cherry tomatoes and cook for 3–5 minutes until softened.
- Serve cod with vegetables and drizzle with fresh lemon juice.

3. Herb-Crusted Salmon with Cucumber-Dill Salad

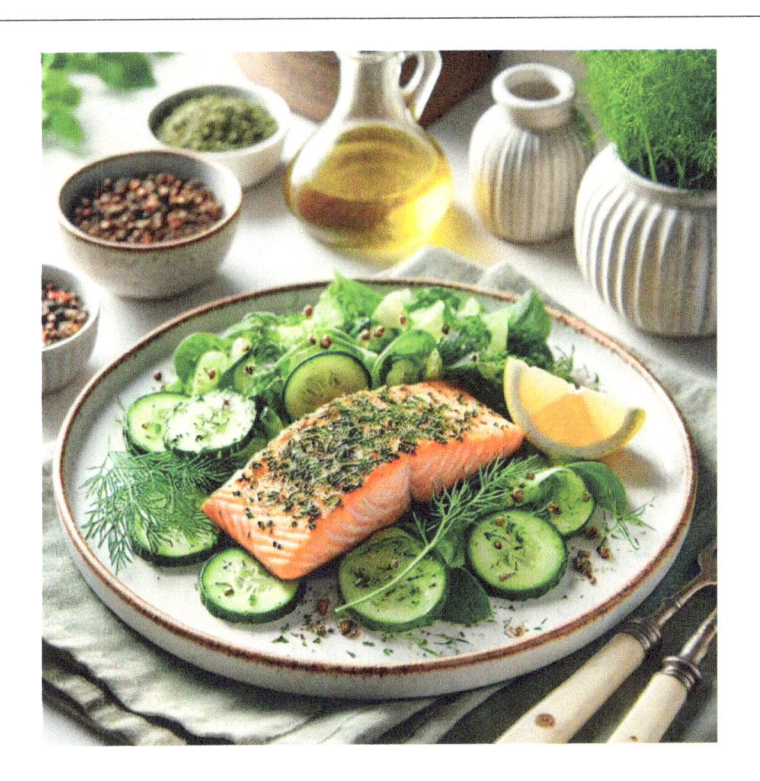

Ingredients:

- 1 wild-caught salmon fillet
- 1 cup sliced cucumbers
- 1 tablespoon fresh dill (chopped)
- 1 tablespoon avocado oil
- ½ teaspoon garlic powder
- ½ teaspoon smoked paprika
- ½ teaspoon Himalayan salt

- Juice of ½ lemon

For Dressing:

- 1 tablespoon olive oil (not heated)
- 1 teaspoon fresh lemon juice
- ½ teaspoon dried dill

Directions:

- Preheat oven to 375°F.
- Pat the fillet dry and rub with garlic powder, smoked paprika, and Himalayan salt for an herb-infused crust.
- Place on a baking sheet and roast for 15–20 minutes until flaky.
- Toss sliced cucumbers and fresh dill in a bowl.
- In a separate small bowl, whisk together olive oil, fresh lemon juice, and dried dill. Drizzle over the cucumber-dill salad.
- Plate the salmon with the fresh salad on the side.

4. Spicy Garlic Chicken with Sautéed Kale and Bell Peppers

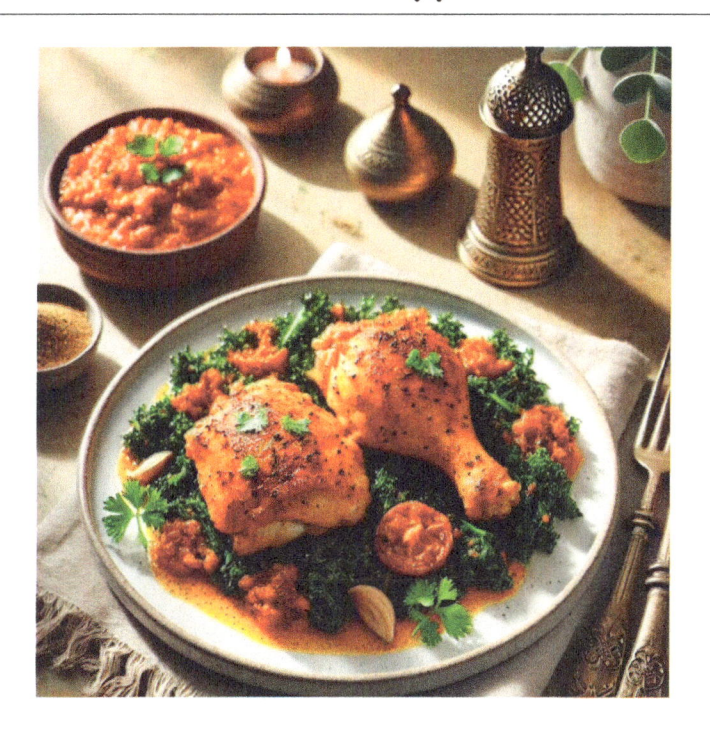

Ingredients:

- 2 chicken thighs (halal optional, skin removed or buy skinless to save time)
- 1 cup chopped kale
- ½ cup sliced bell peppers (mixed colors)
- 1 tablespoon avocado oil
- ½ teaspoon garlic powder
- ½ teaspoon smoked paprika
- ¼ teaspoon cayenne pepper (optional, for heat)

- ½ teaspoon Himalayan salt

Directions:

- Preheat the oven to 375°F.
- Pat dry and rub with garlic powder, smoked paprika, cayenne, and Himalayan salt for bold, spicy flavor.
- Place on a baking sheet and roast for 25–30 minutes until crispy.
- Heat avocado oil in a skillet over medium heat. Add chopped kale and bell peppers and sauté for 3–5 minutes until softened.
- Serve chicken with the sautéed vegetables.

5. Garlic-Lime Chicken with Romaine Lettuce Wraps

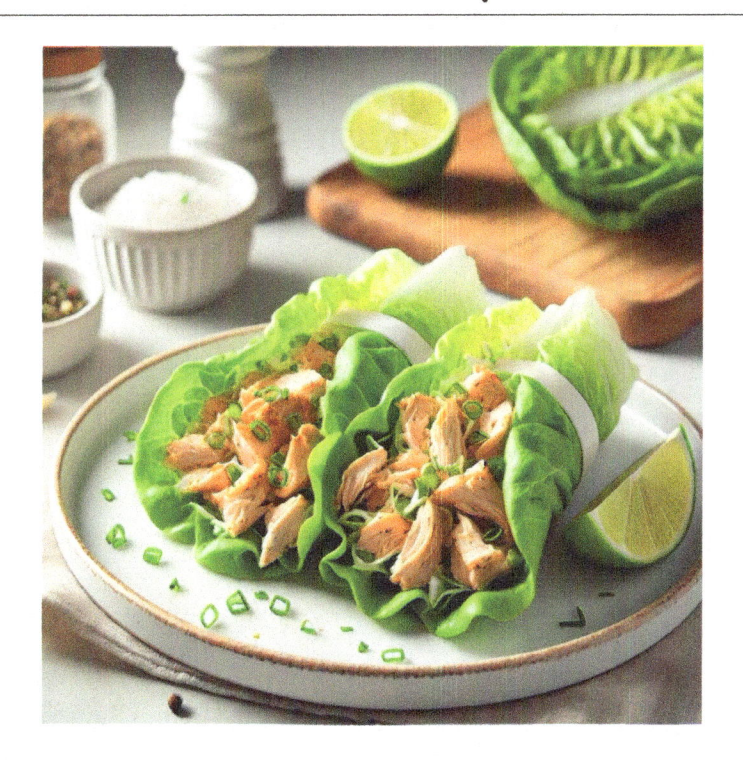

Ingredients:

- 2 chicken thighs (halal optional, skin removed or buy skinless to save time)
- 4 romaine lettuce leaves (whole)
- 1 tablespoon avocado oil
- ½ teaspoon garlic powder
- ½ teaspoon smoked paprika
- ½ teaspoon Himalayan salt

- Juice of ½ lime

Directions:

- Preheat the oven to 375°F.
- Pat the chicken dry and rub with garlic powder, smoked paprika, and Himalayan salt for a deep, flavorful seasoning.
- Place the chicken thighs on a baking sheet and bake for 25–30 minutes until golden and crispy.
- Shred the cooked chicken and place it inside romaine lettuce leaves.
- Drizzle with fresh lime juice before serving.

6. Baked Salmon with Kale and Red Cabbage Slaw

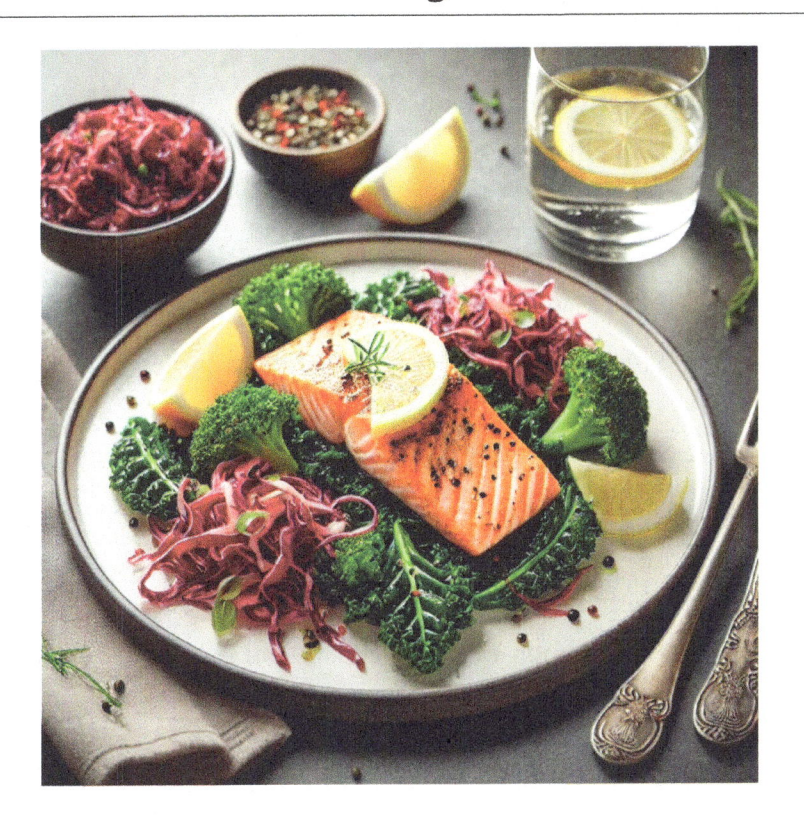

Ingredients:

- 1 wild-caught salmon fillet
- 1 cup chopped kale
- ½ cup shredded red cabbage
- 1 tablespoon avocado oil
- ½ teaspoon garlic powder
- ½ teaspoon Himalayan salt

- Juice of ½ lemon

For Slaw Dressing:

- 1 tablespoon olive oil (not heated)
- 1 teaspoon fresh lemon juice
- 1 teaspoon Dijon mustard

Directions:

- Preheat the oven to 375°F.
- Pat the salmon fillet dry and season with garlic powder and Himalayan salt.
- Place on a baking sheet and bake for 15–20 minutes until flaky.
- Heat avocado oil in a skillet and sauté kale until wilted.
- In a bowl, toss shredded red cabbage with olive oil, lemon juice, and Dijon mustard for a tangy slaw.
- Serve baked salmon with sautéed kale and red cabbage slaw.

7. Basil Lemon Chicken with Sautéed Green Beans and Cherry Tomatoes

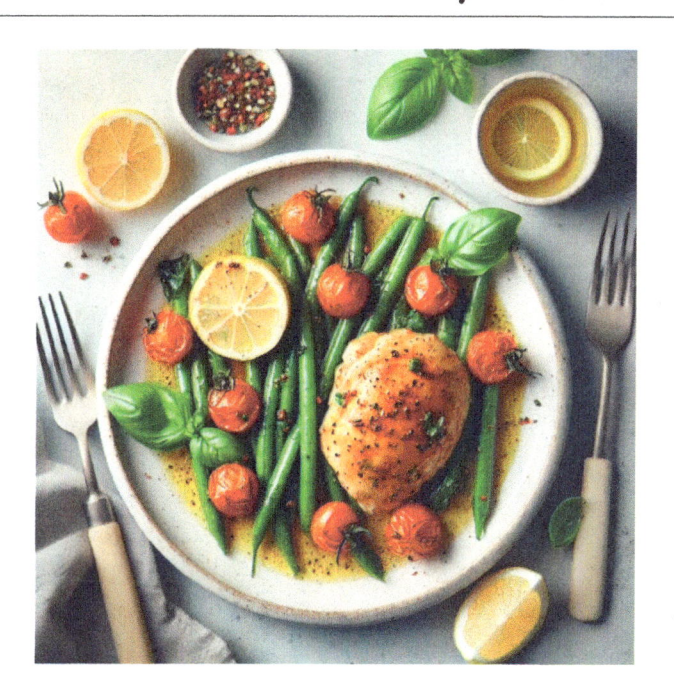

Ingredients:

- 2 chicken thighs (halal optional, skin removed or buy skinless to save time)
- 1 cup green beans
- ½ cup cherry tomatoes (halved)
- 1 tablespoon avocado oil
- ½ teaspoon garlic powder
- ½ teaspoon dried basil
- ½ teaspoon Himalayan salt
- Juice of ½ lemon

Directions:

- Preheat the oven to 375°F.
- Pat the chicken dry and season with garlic powder, dried basil, and Himalayan salt.
- Place on a baking sheet and roast for 25–30 minutes until golden brown.
- Heat avocado oil in a skillet and sauté green beans and cherry tomatoes for 3–5 minutes until tender.
- Serve chicken with vegetables and drizzle with fresh lemon juice.

8. Chicken Thighs with Sautéed Broccoli and Bell Peppers

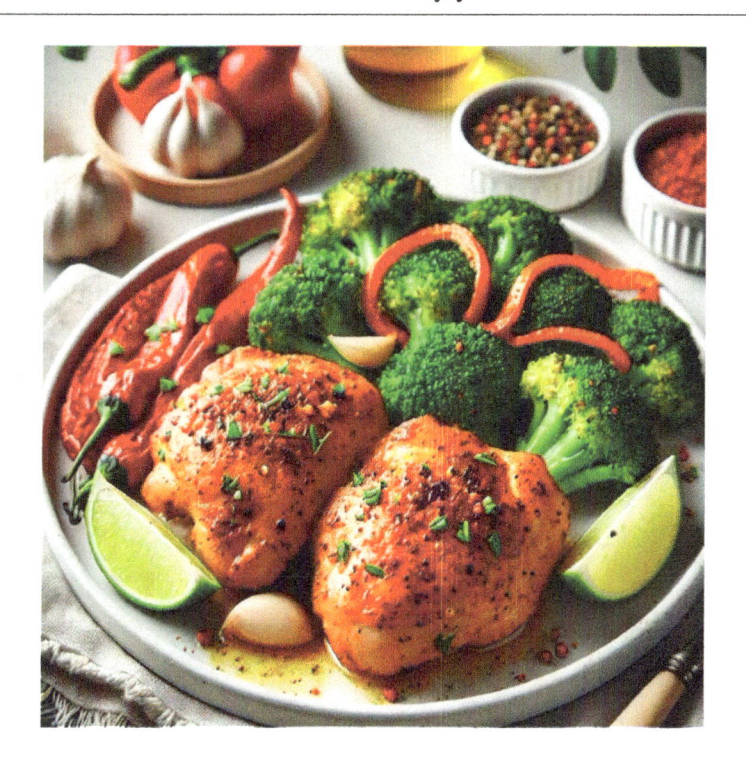

Ingredients:

- 2 chicken thighs (halal optional, skin removed or buy skinless to save time)
- 1 cup broccoli florets
- ½ cup sliced bell peppers (mixed colors)
- 1 tablespoon avocado oil
- ½ teaspoon garlic powder
- ½ teaspoon smoked paprika

- ½ teaspoon Himalayan salt

Directions:

- Preheat the oven to 375°F.
- Pat dry and season the chicken with garlic powder, smoked paprika, and Himalayan salt.
- Place on a baking sheet and roast for 25–30 minutes until golden brown.
- Heat avocado oil in a skillet over medium heat. Add broccoli and bell peppers and sauté for 3–5 minutes until tender.
- Serve chicken with the sautéed vegetables.

9. Zesty Ground Lamb Patties with Fresh Garden Salad

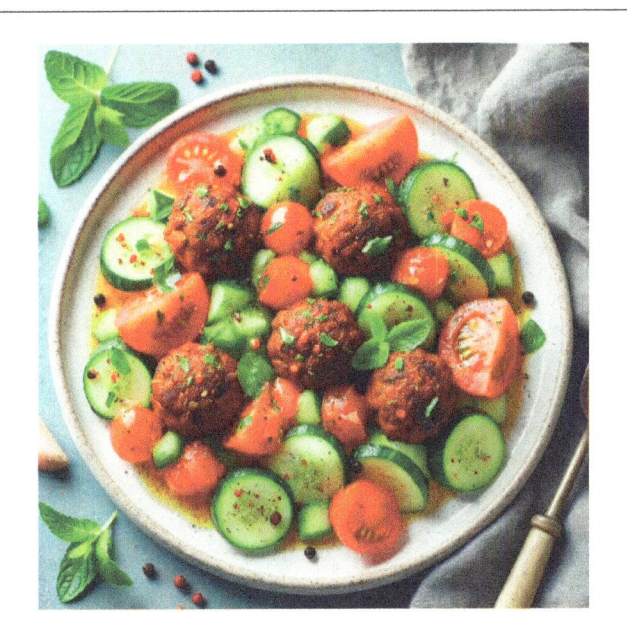

Ingredients for Patties:

- 4 ounces ground lamb (halal optional)
- ½ teaspoon garlic powder
- ½ teaspoon smoked paprika
- ½ teaspoon cumin powder
- ½ teaspoon Himalayan salt

Ingredients for Salad:

- 1 cup chopped romaine lettuce
- ½ cup cherry tomatoes (halved)

- ¼ cup shredded carrots
- ¼ cup sliced cucumber

For Dressing:

- 1 tablespoon olive oil (not heated)
- 1 teaspoon Dijon mustard
- 1 teaspoon fresh lemon juice
- ½ teaspoon garlic powder

Directions:

- Preheat a skillet over medium heat.
- Mix ground lamb with garlic powder, smoked paprika, cumin, and Himalayan salt. Form into two small patties.
- Cook patties in the skillet for 3–4 minutes per side or until fully cooked.
- In a bowl, combine romaine lettuce, cherry tomatoes, carrots, and cucumber.
- In a small bowl, whisk together olive oil, Dijon mustard, lemon juice, and garlic powder for the dressing.
- Drizzle dressing over the salad and serve with lamb patties.

10. Spiced Chicken Salad with Tangy Lemon Dressing

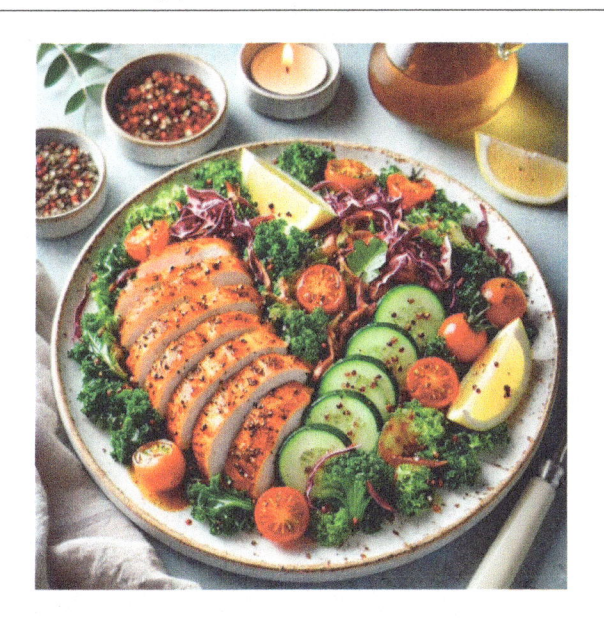

Ingredients for Chicken:

- 2 chicken thighs (halal optional, skin removed or buy skinless to save time)
- ½ teaspoon garlic powder
- ½ teaspoon smoked paprika
- ½ teaspoon Himalayan salt

Ingredients for Salad:

- 1 cup chopped kale
- ½ cup cherry tomatoes (halved)
- ¼ cup shredded red cabbage

- ¼ cup sliced cucumbers

For Dressing:

- 1 tablespoon olive oil (not heated)
- 1 teaspoon Dijon mustard
- Juice of ½ lemon
- ½ teaspoon dried dill

Directions:

- Preheat oven to 375°F.
- Pat dry and season the chicken with garlic powder, smoked paprika, and Himalayan salt.
- Place on a baking sheet and roast for 25–30 minutes or until cooked through.
- In a bowl, combine chopped kale, cherry tomatoes, shredded cabbage, and cucumbers.
- In a small bowl, whisk together olive oil, Dijon mustard, lemon juice, and dried dill for the dressing.
- Slice roasted chicken and place over the salad before serving.

11. Spiced Ground Lamb Patties with Tahini Drizzle and Sautéed Vegetables

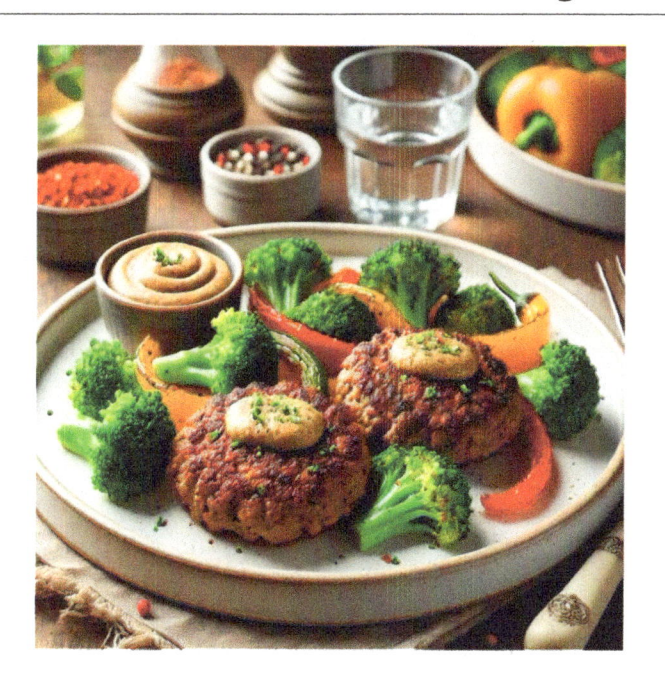

Ingredients for Patties:

- 4 ounces ground lamb (halal optional)
- ½ teaspoon cumin powder
- ½ teaspoon garlic powder
- ½ teaspoon smoked paprika
- ½ teaspoon Himalayan salt

Ingredients for Vegetables:

- 1 cup sautéed broccoli and bell peppers
- ½ teaspoon garlic powder

- 1 teaspoon avocado oil

For Tahini Drizzle:

- 1 tablespoon tahini
- 1 teaspoon fresh lemon juice
- 1 teaspoon water (to thin, if needed)

Directions:

- Preheat a skillet over medium heat.
- Mix ground lamb with cumin, garlic powder, smoked paprika, and Himalayan salt. Form into two small patties.
- Cook patties in the skillet for 3–4 minutes per side or until fully cooked.
- In another skillet, heat avocado oil and sauté broccoli and bell peppers with garlic powder until tender.
- Whisk together tahini, lemon juice, and water to make the drizzle.
- Plate lamb patties with sautéed vegetables and drizzle tahini on top.

12. Lettuce-Wrapped Chicken with Garlic Sauce

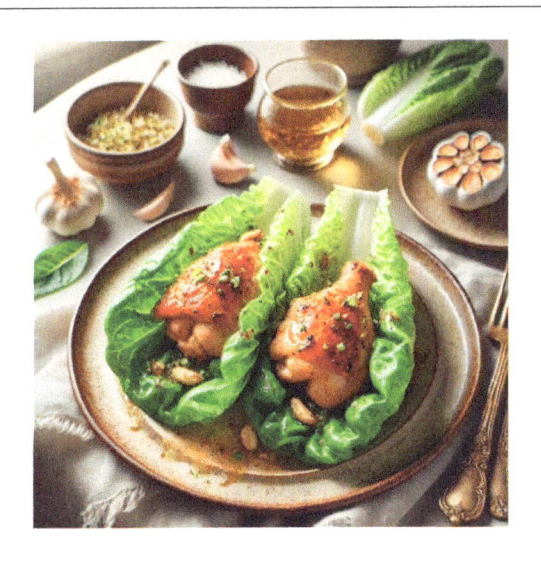

Ingredients for Chicken:

- 2 chicken thighs (halal optional, skin removed or buy skinless to save time)
- ½ teaspoon garlic powder
- ½ teaspoon cumin powder
- ½ teaspoon smoked paprika
- ½ teaspoon Himalayan salt

For Garlic Sauce:

- 1 tablespoon olive oil (not heated)
- 1 teaspoon Dijon mustard
- ½ teaspoon garlic powder

- Juice of ½ lemon

For Wraps:

- 4 large romaine lettuce leaves

Directions:

- Preheat oven to 375°F.
- Pat dry and season the chicken with garlic powder, cumin powder, smoked paprika, and Himalayan salt.
- Place on a baking sheet and roast for 25–30 minutes or until golden brown.
- In a small bowl, whisk together olive oil, Dijon mustard, garlic powder, and lemon juice to make the garlic sauce.
- Slice the chicken and place it in romaine lettuce leaves.
- Drizzle garlic sauce on top and serve.

13. Grilled Chicken Lettuce Wraps with Mango Salsa

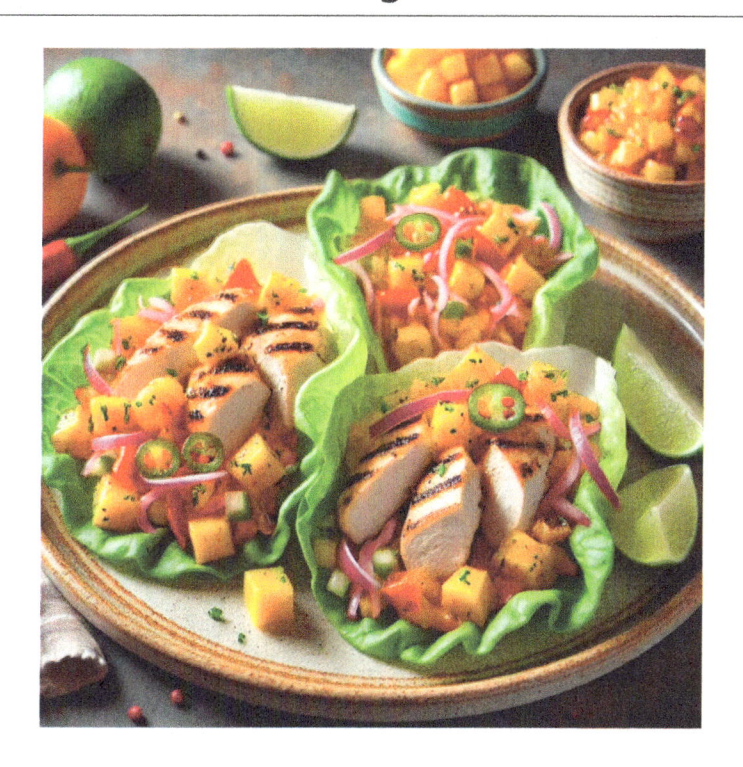

Ingredients for Chicken:

- 2 chicken thighs (halal optional, skin removed or buy skinless to save time)
- ½ teaspoon smoked paprika
- ½ teaspoon garlic powder
- ½ teaspoon cumin powder
- ½ teaspoon Himalayan salt

Ingredients for Mango Salsa:

- ½ cup diced mango
- ¼ cup diced red onion
- ¼ cup diced red bell pepper
- ½ teaspoon lime juice
- 1 small jalapeño, finely diced (optional)

For Wraps:

- 4 large romaine lettuce leaves

Directions:

- Preheat a grill or grill pan.
- Pat dry and season the chicken with smoked paprika, garlic powder, cumin, and Himalayan salt.
- Grill for 5–7 minutes per side or until cooked through.
- In a bowl, combine mango, red onion, red bell pepper, lime juice, and jalapeño for the salsa.
- Slice the grilled chicken and serve in romaine lettuce leaves topped with mango salsa.

Bonus Recipes: Moroccan-Inspired Healing Stews

These nourishing Moroccan stews are packed with flavor, warmth, and nutrient-dense ingredients to support digestion, immunity, and overall well-being. These recipes can be enjoyed as part of your maintenance plan or as a comforting meal anytime.

14. Moroccan Chicken & Vegetable Stew

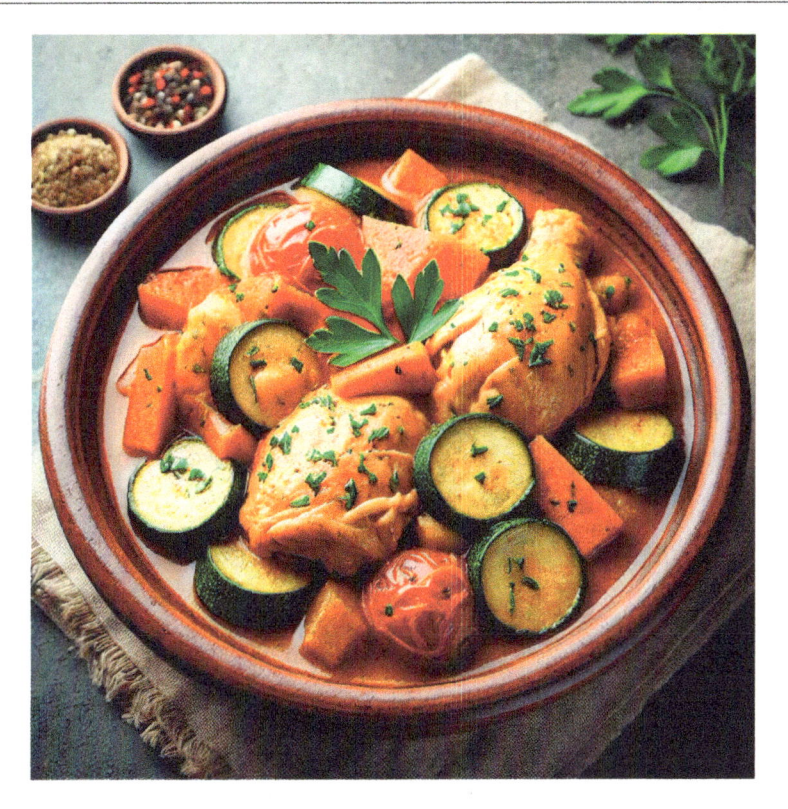

(A warm, aromatic stew with tender chicken, zucchini, and Moroccan spices.)

Ingredients:

- 2 halal chicken thighs (skinless or trimmed of fat)
- 1 cup zucchini, sliced
- ½ cup cherry tomatoes, halved
- ½ cup carrots, chopped
- 1 teaspoon avocado oil

- ½ teaspoon garlic powder
- ½ teaspoon smoked paprika
- ½ teaspoon cumin
- ½ teaspoon turmeric
- ½ teaspoon Himalayan salt
- ½ teaspoon cinnamon (optional, for warmth)
- 1½ cups homemade vegetable broth (or spring water)

Directions:

- Heat avocado oil in a deep pot over medium heat.
- Season the chicken thighs with garlic powder, smoked paprika, cumin, turmeric, and salt.
- Sear the chicken in the pot for 3-4 minutes per side until lightly browned.
- Add carrots, zucchini, and cherry tomatoes, stirring for 2 minutes.
- Pour in vegetable broth and bring to a simmer.
- Cover and let it cook for 25-30 minutes, until the chicken is tender.
- Stir in cinnamon (if using) and let simmer for another 5 minutes.
- Garnish with fresh parsley and serve warm.

Best served on its own for a low-carb option.

15. Moroccan Lamb Meatball & Vegetable Stew

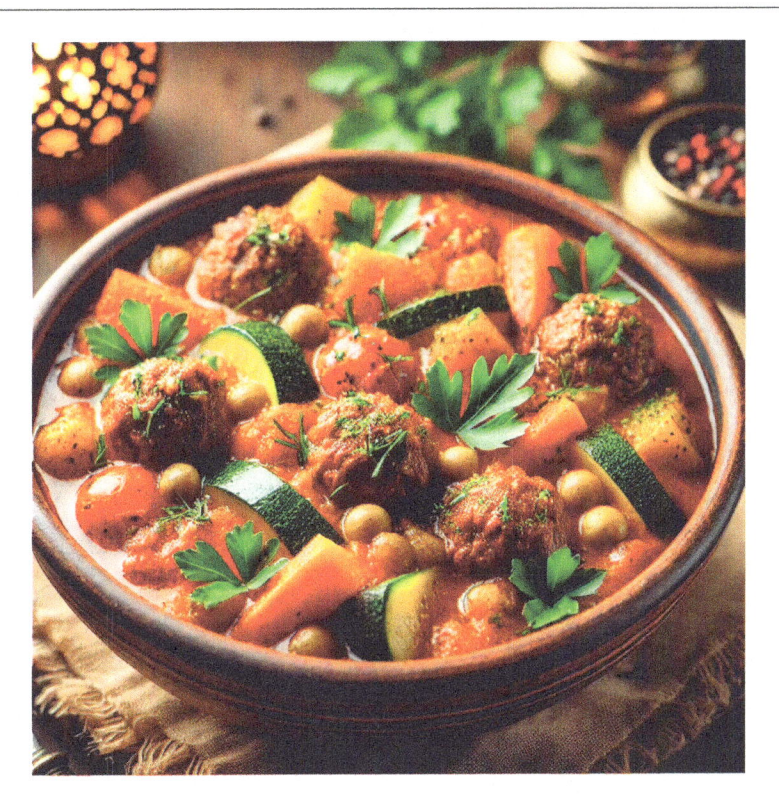

(A rich, spiced dish featuring tender lamb meatballs with zucchini and carrots.)

Ingredients:

- ½ pound halal ground lamb
- ½ teaspoon cumin
- ½ teaspoon smoked paprika
- ½ teaspoon garlic powder

- ½ teaspoon Himalayan salt
- ½ teaspoon turmeric
- 1 tablespoon fresh parsley, chopped
- 1 teaspoon avocado oil
- 1 cup zucchini, chopped
- ½ cup carrots, diced
- ½ cup cherry tomatoes, halved
- 1½ cups homemade vegetable broth

Directions:

- Prepare the meatballs: In a bowl, mix ground lamb, cumin, smoked paprika, garlic powder, Himalayan salt, turmeric, and parsley. Form into small meatballs.
- Heat avocado oil in a deep pan and brown the meatballs for 3-4 minutes per side. Remove and set aside.
- In the same pan, sauté zucchini, carrots, and cherry tomatoes until softened.
- Add vegetable broth, return meatballs to the pan, and let simmer for 15-20 minutes.
- Stir occasionally and let flavors meld.
- Garnish with extra parsley and serve hot.

Best served on its own for a low-carb option.

Why These Recipes Are Special

- Supports digestion with warming spices like cumin, turmeric, and cinnamon.

- Rich in anti-inflammatory ingredients to help reduce bloating and support gut health.
- Balanced protein and fiber to support energy levels and satiety.

Enjoy these bonus recipes anytime for a delicious, healing meal!

Final Notes: Staying Flexible & Adjusting to Your Body

- This plan is a guideline, not a rulebook – Adjust based on your hunger levels and preferences.
- If you're on a budget, swap ingredients for what's affordable – The key is whole, unprocessed foods.
- If you have cravings, increase protein or healthy fats – Adding avocado, nuts, or a bit more protein can help.
- Reach out for support if needed – Email Coach Greg at startyourdetox@gmail.com for adjustments or questions!

What's Next?

Now that you have your full meal plan, let's move into Chapter 6, where you'll learn about how to maintain your results long-term after the detox!

Turn the page to Chapter 6: Post-Detox Maintenance & Lifestyle Plan!

CHAPTER 6

◆ ◆ ◆

Post-Detox Maintenance & Lifestyle Plan

Maintaining Your Results After the 15-Day Reset

Congratulations on completing the Full Body Reset! You've successfully detoxified your body, reduced cravings, and improved your overall well-being. Now, it's time to maintain those results while continuing to enjoy delicious, nourishing meals.

This chapter will cover:

- How to transition back to regular meals while maintaining your progress.
- Which foods to reintroduce and which to limit or avoid.
- The importance of juicing & investing in a cold-pressed juicer.
- How to use supplements daily for long-term benefits.
- The best salads & homemade dressings to bring variety to your meals.
- Mushroom-based burgers & plant-based alternatives.
- The role of slow cookers & pressure cookers for meal prep.
- How Japanese yams naturally sweeten greens.
- A new food pyramid tailored for long-term health.

Reintroducing Foods Without Losing Progress

As you transition from detox mode, slowly add back foods one at a time every 3-4 days. This helps you understand how your body reacts and prevents bloating, sluggishness, or cravings.

Smart Carbs for Long-Term Health

- Quinoa (A high-protein grain, easy to digest.)
- Basmati Rice (Lower glycemic, better for digestion.)
- Cauliflower Rice (Great low-carb alternative.)
- Chickpea Pasta or Brown Rice Pasta (Avoid regular wheat pasta.)
- Sprouted Bread (Frozen Section) (Options: Ezekiel, sprouted bagels, English muffins, toast.)

High-Quality Proteins

- Wild-Caught Fish (Pole-Caught Tuna, Salmon, Cod, Mahi-Mahi) (Always in water with sea salt.)
- Pasture-Raised Eggs (If Tolerated)
- Organic, Pasture-Raised Chicken & Turkey
- Grass-Fed Beef or Lamb (Moderation Only)
- Mushroom-Based Burgers (Portobello, Shiitake, or Oyster Mushrooms as a Meat Alternative)

Healthy Fats

- Avocado & Avocado Mayo (For sandwiches & wraps.)
- Olive Oil & Coconut Oil (For cooking & salads.)

- Raw Nuts & Seeds (Almonds, Walnuts, Flaxseeds, Chia Seeds) (Nutrient-dense & anti-inflammatory.)

Fermented & Gut-Healing Foods

- Kimchi & Sauerkraut (Supports digestion & gut health.)
- Pickles (Raw, Brine-Fermented) (Boosts probiotics, avoid vinegar-based.)
- Coconut Yogurt or Kefir (Dairy-Free Option) (Great for gut health.)

Best Sauces & Condiments

- Coconut Aminos (A low-sodium soy sauce alternative.)
- Dijon Mustard (No added sugar.)
- *Homemade Dressings (Olive Oil, Lemon, Herbs, Spices.)

What to Avoid (or Limit for Best Results)

- Processed Sugar (Causes cravings & energy crashes.)
- Refined Carbs (White Bread, Pasta, Processed Grains) (Increases bloating & weight gain.)
- Dairy (If Sensitive) (May cause bloating, acne, congestion.)
- Seed Oils (Canola, Vegetable, Soybean, Corn Oil) (Inflammatory.)
- Fast Food & Packaged Snacks (Contains preservatives, unhealthy fats, hidden sugars.)

The Power of Juicing: Why Invest in a Cold-Pressed Juicer?

Juicing is one of the fastest ways to flood your body with vitamins, minerals, and hydration. A cold-pressed juicer ensures you get the highest nutrient retention without damaging enzymes.

Juicing Benefits & What to Juice for Specific Needs

- Cantaloupe Juice – Hydration & Bowel Regularity (High in water & electrolytes, supports digestion.)
- Watermelon & Beet Juice – Energy Boost (Increases circulation, oxygenates the blood.)
- Apples, Grapes & Mint – Refreshing & Tasty (Great for detoxing and flavor balance.)
- Pineapple-Ginger-Apple Juice – Digestion Support (Reduces bloating, soothes the gut.)

If buying store-bought juice, choose organic, unfiltered options like Dole 100% Pineapple Juice or non-concentrate brands.

Building the Perfect Salad: Make It Exciting!

Salads should never feel like a boring "diet" food. The key is variety, texture, and a great dressing.

Salad Base Options (Choose 1-2 Greens Per Salad)

- Romaine, Kale, Arugula, Spinach, Red Leaf Lettuce, Butter Lettuce

Add a Crunch (Choose 1-2)

- Cucumber, Bell Peppers, Red Cabbage, Carrots, Pickles

Healthy Proteins (Choose 1)

- Grilled Chicken, Wild-Caught Fish, Ground Lamb, Boiled Egg (If Tolerated), Mushroom-Based Patties

Dressing Ideas (Easy & Homemade!)

- Avocado Ranch: Blend avocado, olive oil, garlic powder, lemon juice, fresh dill.
- Dairy-Free Blue Cheese: Blend cashew butter, Dijon mustard, apple cider vinegar, garlic powder.

How to Use a Slow Cooker or Pressure Cooker for Easy Meals

- Slow Cookers (Crockpots): Great for overnight stews, lamb, chicken, or lentils without constant monitoring.
- Pressure Cookers (Instant Pots): Cuts cooking time in half and locks in flavor—perfect for making quinoa, lentils, and stews fast!

Tip: Cooking collard greens with Japanese yams in a pressure cooker naturally sweetens them without sugar!

How to Use Supplements Daily for Long-Term Health

High School Skinny – Take every morning to control cravings & maintain fat loss.

- Blue Shield – 2x per week for circulation & inflammation support.
- Full Battery – Take daily for energy & avoiding sluggishness.

- Stress Free Genius – 3-4x per week for relaxation, mental clarity, & deep sleep.
- Green Multi – 3-4x per week for essential minerals & muscle recovery.

EvenTone Skin, Pressure Balance, and Milk Silk Cream should be continued as needed based on results.

Final Words: This Is Just the Beginning!

You've worked hard—now enjoy the results and live your healthiest life!

- Eat in a way that fuels your body.
- Experiment with salads, juices, and homemade meals.
- Listen to your body and adjust as needed.
- Keep using your supplements daily for best results!

Don't Forget to Leave a Review!

Your feedback matters! If you've enjoyed the program, please leave a review on the supplements and products.

For questions or support, reach out to Coach Greg at startyourdetox@gmail.com.

CHAPTER 7

◆ ◆ ◆

Healing Recipes for Vitamin & Mineral Deficiencies & Common Health Concerns

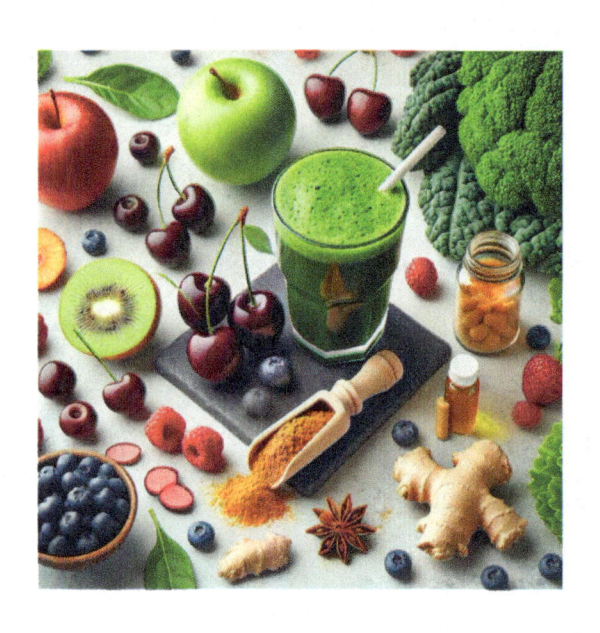

Using Food to Restore Nutrient Balance & Improve Health Naturally

Many health concerns—from skin issues and low energy to high cholesterol and digestive problems—are caused by vitamin and mineral deficiencies or imbalances in the body.

This chapter includes:

- What deficiencies cause certain health issues
- Foods rich in those missing nutrients
- Healing recipes to restore balance
- Supplement recommendations for faster results
- FAQs to answer your most common questions

Healing Recipes for Health Concerns

1. Dark Spots Under Eyes & Skin Issues

EvenTone Skin & Green Multi

Healing Green Juice

- 1 small green apple
- ½ cup kale
- ½ cup green grapes
- 6 fresh mint leaves
- 1 cup spring water
- Add 1 tablespoon EvenTone Skin & 1 tablespoon Blue Shield

2. Cellulite & Wrinkles

EvenTone Skin & Green Multi

Citrus Collagen Smoothie

- 1 cup frozen mango
- ½ cup fresh pineapple
- 1 tablespoon chia seeds
- ½ teaspoon turmeric
- 1 cup coconut water
- Add 1 tablespoon EvenTone Skin & 1 tablespoon Green Multi

3. Brittle Nails & Hair Loss

Hair Food & Green Multi

Berry Beauty Smoothie

- ½ cup frozen blueberries
- ½ cup frozen raspberries
- 1 tablespoon flaxseeds
- 1 teaspoon maca powder
- 1 cup almond or coconut milk
- Add 1 tablespoon Hair Food & 1 tablespoon Green Multi

4. High Cholesterol

Blue Shield & Green Multi (Cholesterol drops 30 points in 2 weeks!)

Cherry Berry Cholesterol-Lowering Smoothie

- 1 cup frozen dark cherries
- ½ cup frozen raspberries
- 1 teaspoon chia seeds
- 1 teaspoon flaxseeds
- 1 cup spring water
- Add 1 tablespoon Green Multi & 1 tablespoon Blue Shield

5. Bloating & Slow Digestion

High School Skinny

Berry Detox Smoothie

- 1 cup frozen dark sweet cherries
- ½ cup frozen raspberries
- 2 tablespoons High School Skinny
- 1 cup spring water

6. Moles & Candida Overgrowth

High School Skinny & Blue Shield

Anti-Candida Tonic

- 1 teaspoon apple cider vinegar
- ½ teaspoon turmeric powder
- ½ teaspoon grated ginger
- 1 teaspoon lemon juice
- 1 cup spring water

FULL BODY RESET

- Add 1 tablespoon High School Skinny & 1 tablespoon Blue Shield

7. Insomnia & Poor Sleep

Stress Free Genius

Sleepy Time Smoothie

- ½ frozen banana
- 1 teaspoon flaxseeds
- ½ teaspoon cinnamon
- 1 cup almond milk
- Add 1 tablespoon Stress Free Genius

8. Cold & Mucus Congestion

Blue Shield

Pineapple Mucus Cleanser

- 1 cup Dole 100% Pineapple Juice
- ½ teaspoon grated ginger
- ½ teaspoon cayenne pepper
- Add 2 tablespoons Blue Shield

9. Muscle & Joint Weakness

Green Multi & Full Battery

Pineapple Muscle Recovery Juice

- 1 cup Dole 100% Pineapple Juice
- ½ teaspoon turmeric

- ½ teaspoon ginger
- ½ teaspoon cinnamon
- Add 1 tablespoon Green Multi & 1 tablespoon Full Battery

FAQs (Frequently Asked Questions)

How long should I continue using the supplements after the detox?

Use daily for best results.

What if I miss a day of supplements?

Resume the next day—no need to double up.

Can I keep drinking the detox smoothies and juices daily?

Yes! Many continue drinking ABC Juice, green juices, and smoothies for long-term benefits.

Can I swap ingredients if I have allergies?

Yes! Example swaps:
- Pineapple → Mango
- Nuts → Seeds

Can I drink coffee?

No. Double the dosage of Full Battery to 2 tablespoons instead.

How long before I see results?

- Skin, digestion, and sleep improve by Day 5.

- Energy improves by Day 1-2. Full Battery works very fast.
- Weight loss is daily. Don't be afraid of the scale—numbers don't lie.
- Cholesterol improves by the end of 15 days.
- Sleep improves the same day.

What's the best time to take my supplements?

- Morning: High School Skinny, Full Battery, Green Multi
- Afternoon: Blue Shield, EvenTone Skin
- Night: Stress Free Genius (for sleep)

Do I need a juicer?

Cold-pressed juicers are best, but blending & straining also works.

What's the best store-bought juice?

- Dole 100% Pineapple Juice (No added sugar.)
- Unfiltered Organic Apple Juice

How often should I do the Full Body Reset?

Every 4 months or twice a year for a full system reboot!

For questions, reach out to Coach Greg at startyourdetox@gmail.com

CHAPTER 8

◆ ◆ ◆

Closing Remarks & Gratitude

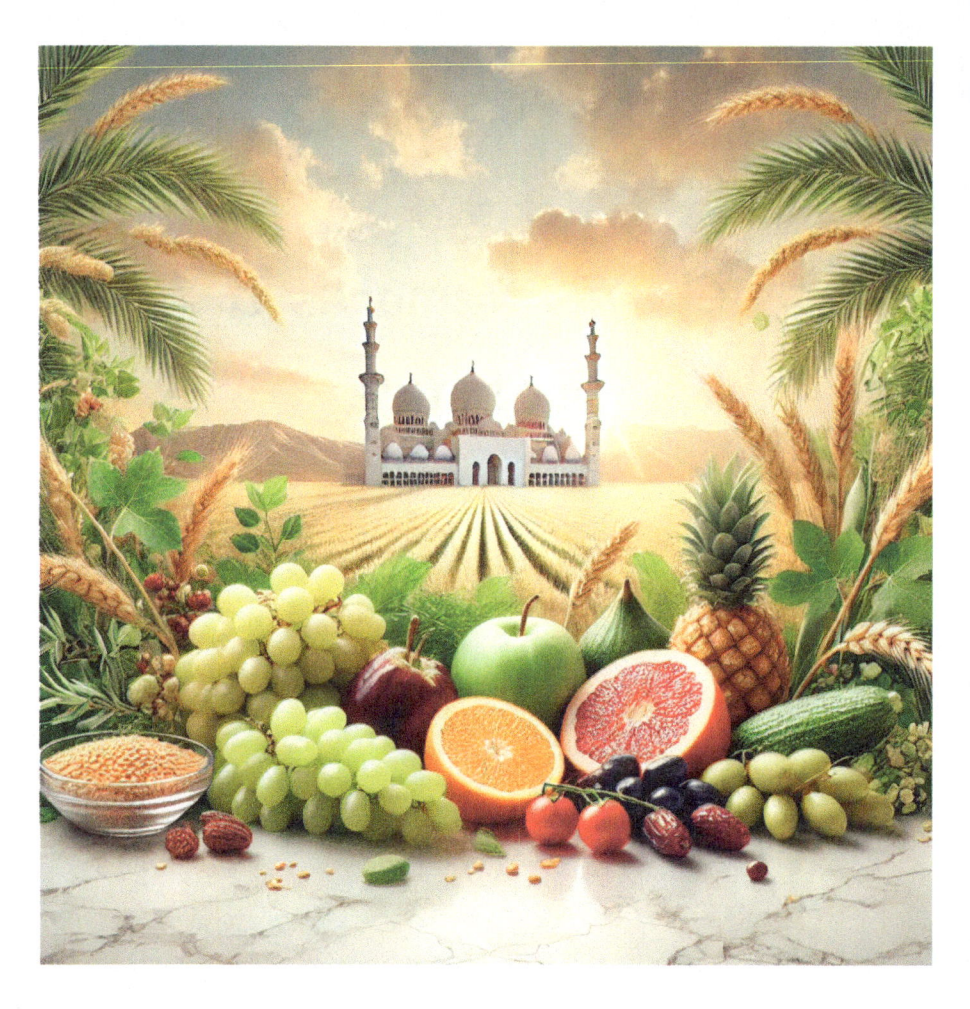

Giving Thanks for Health & Guidance

As we reach the end of this journey, we must acknowledge that true health, healing, and strength come only by the mercy and guidance of Allah. The foods we consume, the ability to cleanse and renew our bodies, and even the knowledge to make better choices—all are blessings from Him.

Allah has created every cure in nature, providing us with the foods that nourish, heal, and restore balance. Our responsibility is to honor these blessings by taking care of our bodies, staying mindful of what we consume, and striving to live a life of wellness, clarity, and discipline.

Reflection on the Blessings of Food in the Quran

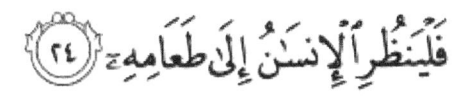

$$\text{فَلْيَنظُرِ ٱلْإِنسَٰنُ إِلَىٰ طَعَامِهِۦٓ ۝}$$

Let Man consider his nourishment.

$$\text{أَنَّا صَبَبْنَا ٱلْمَآءَ صَبًّا ۝}$$

We send down abundant water.

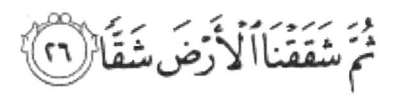

$$\text{ثُمَّ شَقَقْنَا ٱلْأَرْضَ شَقًّا ۝}$$

And We split the earth in fragments

$$\text{فَأَنۢبَتْنَا فِيهَا حَبًّا ۝}$$

And caused to grow within it grain

$$\text{وَعِنَبًا وَقَضْبًا ۝}$$

And Grapes and nutritious plants

$$\text{وَزَيْتُونًا وَنَخْلًا ﴿٢٩﴾}$$

And olive-trees and palm-trees

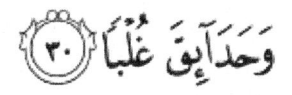

$$\text{وَحَدَائِقَ غُلْبًا ﴿٣٠﴾}$$

And gardens, dense with many trees

$$\text{وَفَاكِهَةً وَأَبًّا ﴿٣١﴾}$$

And fruits and herbage

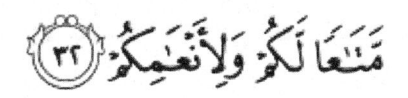

$$\text{مَتَاعًا لَكُمْ وَلِأَنْعَامِكُمْ ﴿٣٢﴾}$$

Provision for you and your cattle.

Quran
Chapter 80
Verses 24-32

These verses remind us that every bite we take is a sign of Allah's mercy. He has made food grow from the earth, nourished by water, to sustain us. This is why we must be grateful and intentional in what we eat—choosing natural, pure, and wholesome foods that align with the way our bodies were created.

A Journey, Not Just a Detox

This program was never about a temporary cleanse—it's about learning to live in a way that honors your body, your mind, and your purpose.

- Continue making mindful food choices.
- Stay disciplined in your habits.
- Use the knowledge you've gained to help others.
- Remember that true health begins with gratitude and intention.

The journey to better health does not end here. Each day is a new opportunity to improve, to seek balance, and to strengthen your connection with the natural provisions Allah has blessed us with.

Final Words: A Life of Wellness & Purpose

- Take what you've learned and apply it daily.
- Share this knowledge with your family and loved ones.
- Remember that true wellness is physical, mental, and spiritual.
- Keep striving for better, knowing that Allah has provided everything you need to thrive.

May Allah bless you with good health, strength, and clarity. May He continue to guide you towards the best choices for your body and your soul.

Alhamdulillah for everything.

Eyes Tell All Detox Club

For media inquiries, or to contact Coach Greg for speaking engagements, health consultations, general questions and school events, email: StartYourDetox@gmail.com

Made in the USA
Coppell, TX
14 May 2025

49287295R00049